Anti Inflammatory Diet:

Best Healthy Recipes to Help Yourself

Table of content

Introduction

Health is wealth! That saying is just as true today as it was several hundred years ago. Health is the most crucial factor in the life of an individual. A healthy living in today's world has become rather challenging due to fast-paced routines and the trend of processed foods. Adults and children alike have utterly busy schedules and cannot accommodate exercise or pay attention to nutrition. However, if the benefits of a healthy life were to be compared with the efforts required to follow healthy habits, the advantages would far outweigh the efforts and are extremely beneficial in the long run.

In this book, we perform in-depth exploration of topics like inflammation, immunity and brain health. Furthermore, you will learn natural and organic ways to treat and prevent such problems without the unwelcome intervention of medicine that cast several side effects on your health. We have listed and discussed foods that can aid you in boosting and promoting the natural defense mechanisms of your body. Incorporating these in your diet will not only ensure the proper functioning of your bodily and cognitive function but will also increase your natural immune response by enabling your body to adapt to natural resources and tackling problems in a natural manner.

Health being the most fundamental factor of a satisfactory life, evidently, it seems sensible to make choices that benefit your health. So embark with us on this journey as we explore how to take good care of your body by tackling problems related to inflammation, immunity and mind while avoiding unnecessary and harmful medication using all natural resources and your body will thank you!

Chapter 1 – Anti Inflammatory Diet to Avoid Medication

A person's diet has the largest impact on the overall health of the body. A poor, unbalanced diet can lead to inflammation of the gut. Foods rich in processed carbohydrates, fried food, carbonated drinks in excess amounts etcetera serve to facilitate diet induced inflammation. If not attended to or taken care of, inflammation becomes a very tedious and chronic problem.

There are multiple ways that one can employ to altogether avoid inflammation. One of the most increasingly popular ways that have come to light in the recent past to avoid inflammation is the use of diet that is absolutely anti-inflammatory. The diet is strictly exclusive of food items that promote inflammation and generally promotes adding those foods to your daily diet plan that have innate anti-inflammatory properties. The table below illustrates few of the food categories, their source and their benefit in anti-inflammatory diet.

Table 1. Tabular summary of foods possessing anti-inflammatory properties

Category	Source	Benefit
Fruits and vegetables	Green leafy vegetables, red fruits like berries	Rich in anti-oxidants
Whole grains	Unrefined wheat, brown rice, lentils	Rich in fiber, low in carbohydrates. No added sugar.
Low fat dairy	Skimmed Milk, Yogurt	Essential nutrients, probiotic
Lean protein	Chicken and Fish such as salmon, herring, black cod, sardines	Rich in Omega 3 fatty acids.
Essential fats	Olive oil, nut butters (cashews, almonds, peanuts)	Healthy nutrients essential for balanced diet

Generally speaking, diet consisting of fruits and vegetables, lean proteins and whole grains has an anti-inflammatory effect. Each of these aforementioned foods are discussed in brief detail as follows.

Fruits and Vegetables

In order to have a proper and balanced diet, the incorporation of fresh fruits and vegetables is highly recommended. Inflammation in the general sense is caused by pro inflammatory molecules called *cytokines*. Vegetables such green leafy ones are rich in vitamin E which fights to protect the body from cytokines that promote inflammation. The best sources of this vitamin are dark green vegetables such as spinach, kale and broccoli among others.

Almost all fruits and vegetables help fight inflammation since they are known to possess low levels of fats and calories and comparatively elevated levels of antioxidants which helps fight inflammation. Amongst fruits, berries are richest source of antioxidants and hence have anti-inflammatory properties. It is suggested that berries owe their properties to the presence of a chemical called *anthocyanins* that also give berries their rich red color.

Scientific evidence exhibits that blueberries provide a natural defense against intestinal inflammation. A study showed that animals who were given red raspberry extract aided them in prevention of the development of arthritis. In 2012, a study conducted at Oregon Health and Science University stated that cherries had the most anti-inflammatory properties out of all the fruits and vegetables. It is suggested that they even help inflammation pain hence reducing the intake of pain management medicine making it a great natural preventive measure. Moreover, pungent vegetables like onions, ginger and garlic are popular due to the presence of anti-inflammatory chemicals like phytonutrient quercetin that fights inflammation.

Whole grains

Consumption of whole grains as opposed to that of processed ones is highly recommended for not just anti-inflammatory but a healthy diet in general. Whole grains such as wheat, barely, maize, corn, rice and lentils are rich in fiber and low in carbohydrates. In contrast, processed grains have a high carbohydrate content which poses health risks. Reducing your intake of refined foods will aid in keeping inflammation at bay. As an added advantage, these unprocessed, high fiber whole grains have no added sugar which is a plus for weight watchers.

Low fat dairy

Low fat dairy products like milk and yogurt are a rich source of a multiple variety of essential nutrients that help maintain a balanced diet. Yogurt is a natural probiotic which means that it contains helpful bacteria that aid your digestion and keeps your gut on track while fighting harmful infection. This natural probiotic not only fights infection but also aids in fighting inflammation of the gut. Yogurt and skim milk have also been shown to help the inflammation caused by rheumatoid arthritis.

Lean protein and healthy fats

Lean protein such as white meat including fish and chicken forms a necessary component of anti-inflammatory nutrition plan. Avoiding red meats which are pro inflammatory can reduce risk of inflammation. Healthy fats such as omega 3 fatty acids in fish are pro health. Avoid eating butter, vegetable oils such as sunflower and corn and incorporate olive oil in your diet which is much healthier and safer option. It is also gentle on the heart.

Incorporating all the aforementioned food items in your daily diet can considerably help intercept inflammation as well as alleviate its symptoms in a natural and organic way without the intervention of western medicine that poses myriad side effects. It is highly advised to include these items in your diet so as to prevent inflammation. As the saying goes, prevention is better than cure.

Chapter 2 – Diet to Improve Body Immunity

Understanding Immunity

The human body is a complicated system comprising of several intricate mechanisms that need to work together in harmony in order to make up a healthy human. Amongst them, a system that is fundamental to physical wellbeing of an individual is the immune system. Immune system is actually a group of mechanisms in the body that help the body fight against any intruders. In simpler words, the immune system is the body's natural defense against disease. It fights all foreign agents hence defending the body against any outside invasion. When a foreign agent such as a bacteria or a virus enters the body, the immune system becomes activated and tries to harm it before it can start causing harm to the body. If, due to some reason, the body's immune system is compromised, the body becomes defenseless and extremely susceptible to disease causing bacteria and viruses which in severe cases can eventually result in fatality. Therefore, in order to stay healthy, it is of foremost importance that the immune system stays 100% efficient.

Foods to Aid Immunity

The best way to ensure and boost immunity is to provide your body with natural immunity boosting foods. Certain foods that have been known to improve immunity can be incorporated in your diet. These natural products have no harmful side effects as opposed to their medicinal counterparts and are a beneficial and natural way of promoting the body's natural defense against disease. Some such foods are discussed as follows.

- *Herbs*

    Herbs are a great way to boost your immunity in a natural way. Some examples of herbs that have been popularly used for boosting your natural defense are *Echinacea, Ginseng, Astragalus, Cats's claw* among others. These herbs can be taken as tea or sprinkled dried or fresh over any dish not only improving taste but also invigorate immunity as an added benefit. The table below lists the individual advantages of these herbs.

Table 2. Herbs and their uses in improving immunity

Herb	Benefit
Echinacea	Prevents and treats respiratory infection & common cold
Ginseng	Anti-inflammatory & anti-cancer benefits.
Astragalus	Rich in flavonoids. Aids digestions, promotes immunity, prevents and treats cold and flu
Cat's claw	Aids immunity by promoting response to infection. Source of oxindole alkaloids which helps the body in destroying pathogens
Oregano	Rich in carvacrol and thymol which have anti-bacterial, anti-fungal and anti-virus properties. Helps flush intestinal parasites
Peppermint	Rich in menthol that inhibits bacterial growth

- *Spices*

Much like herbs, spices are also a great source of chemical compounds that facilitate defense mechanisms of the body. Some examples and their benefits have been elaborated in the table below.

Table 3. Spices that boost immunity

Spice	Benefit
Turmeric	Boosts immunity by preventing neuro degenerative diseases, cancer, diabetes. Natural painkiller.
Cinnamon	Lowers risk of diabetes, aids cancer treatment, inhibits microbial growth
Cayenne	Boosts metabolism, fights cancer, anti-inflammatory properties

- *Grains*

Grains form an essential part of a balanced diet. When taken in unprocessed and unrefined state they provide us with numerous benefits. Not only are they a great source of fiber but they also simultaneously aid the body's natural defense against harmful disease causing agents. Grains like oats and barely have been known to improve immunity. Both these grains are a rich source of a compound called beta-glucan. In accordance to a Norwegian study, this compound possess antimicrobial and antioxidant properties. When tested on animals, the results exhibited that the subjects were much less probable to infections like influenza and herpes. In humans, oats and barely have been shown to boost defense by aiding antibiotics.

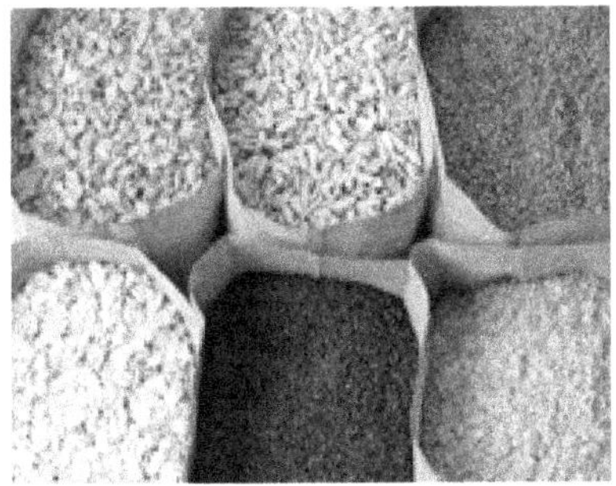

http://www.newsnish.com/wp-content/uploads/2015/06/download-6.jpg

* *Yogurt*

It is a known fact that the health benefits of yogurt are tenfold. It is the most popular probiotic. That basically just implies that it contains live cultures of healthy bacteria. These bacteria provide health benefits by keeping harmful disease causing germs at bay and keeping the intestinal tract free of any harmful bacteria hence promoting immunity.

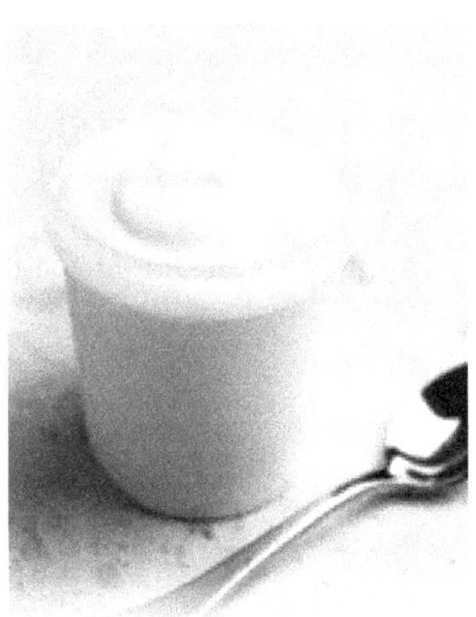

https://belikewaterproduction.files.wordpress.com/2014/07/yogurt.jpg?w=250&h=300

* *Healthy Meats*

One of the greatest sources of white meats is fish. Fish such as salmon, and mackerel are both widely known great sources of omega 3 fatty acids which are known to prevent and treat lung and respiratory infections. Moreover, chicken can also boost immunity since while cooking, it releases chemicals similar to respiratory infection drug *acetyl cysteine* which better prepares your body for fighting infection as well as aids cold treatment.

Apart from white meats, beef is also known to aid defense due to being a rich source of the mineral zinc. The presence of zinc in your diet is extremely crucial to the synthesis of white blood cells which are functioning unit of the body's immune response to infection. These cells are responsible for recognizing and destroying foreign agents such as bacteria and viruses hence facilitating defense.

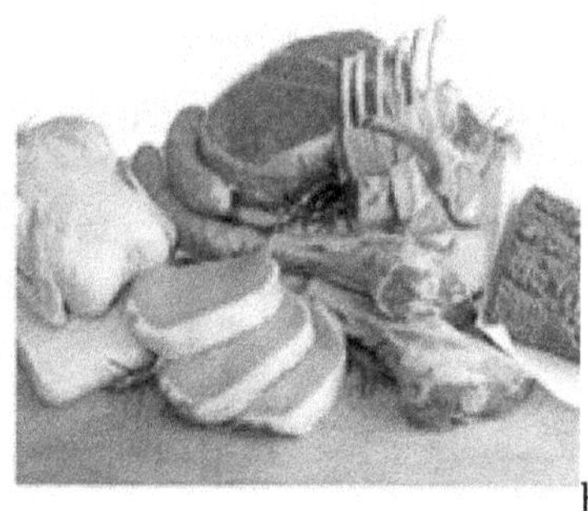

http://www.mesara-minjon-d.com/ images/mes01.jpg

Chapter 3 – Treat your inflammation with food items

Inflammation being a common problem has a lot of medicinal treatment options. But the usage of western medicine comes at a huge price. Not only does it house in itself multitude side effects but also aims to lower your body's natural ability to fight so the body becomes addicted to medicine and hence fails to work itself out even when the problem is fairly simple. A great way to avoid this is to incorporate home remedies consisting of foods that you may include in your diet to naturally treat inflammation. Some such options are discussed in this chapter.

What to eat?

Healthy oils

One of foremost causes of inflammation includes excessive use of unhealthy fat in your diet. It is advised to substitute vegetable oils like sunflower and corn for healthier options such as olive oil or avocado oil. These oils are not only great tasting but also aid treat and prevent inflammation. Olive oil is a rich source of oleic and omega-3 fatty acids which is what is meant by "good fats". They aid the decrease in inflammation.

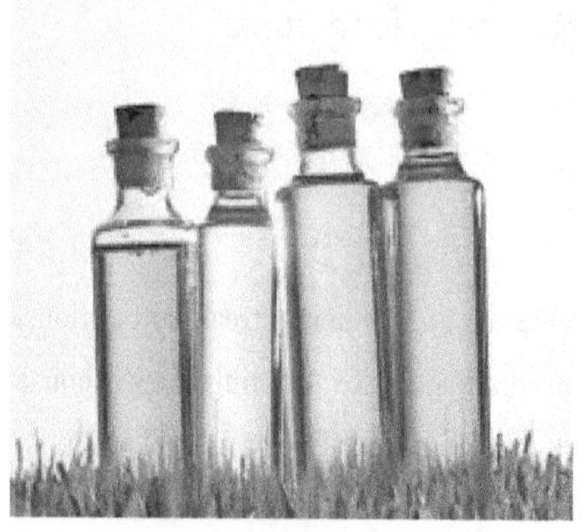

http://naturalmentor.com/wp-content/uploads/2015/11/healthyoils.jpg

Pro-biotics

Products containing live bacterial cultures of good bacteria are a very beneficial remedy for inflammation. Fermented products like yogurt and soft cheeses are particularly high sources of live cultures. The bacteria present in these cultures fight the harmful microbes in the digestive tract hence soothing and treating inflammation.

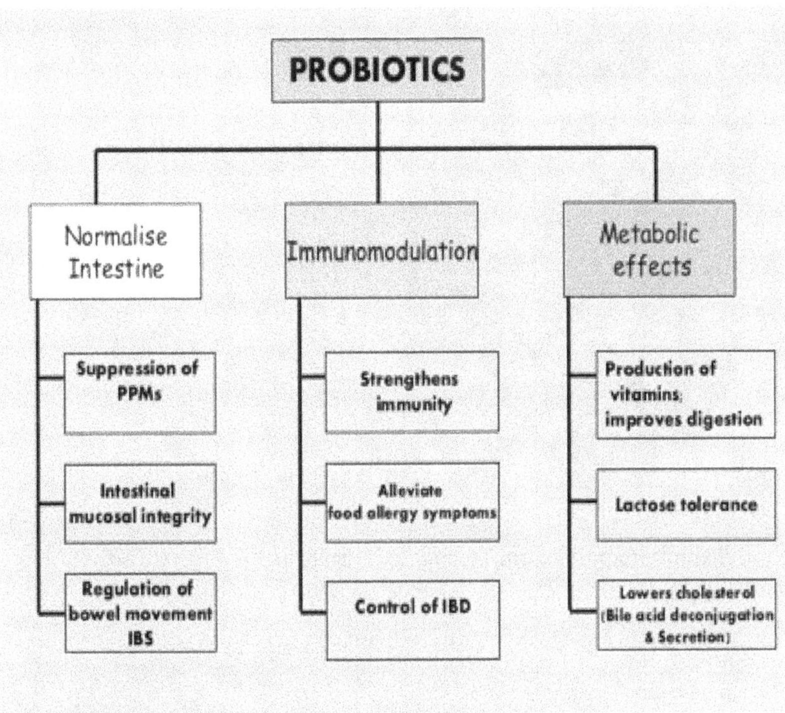

http://image.slidesharecdn.com/preprobiotics-141014183151-conversion-gate01/95/prebiotics-and-probiotics-22-638.jpg?cb=1413311663

Dry fruits

Dried fruits and nuts such as walnuts, almonds, cashews and peanuts are all rich sources of antioxidants. The antioxidant compounds present in these nuts make them a prime food item that aids the treatment of inflammation in a natural manner. The antioxidants fight the free radicals that cause inflammation in the body.

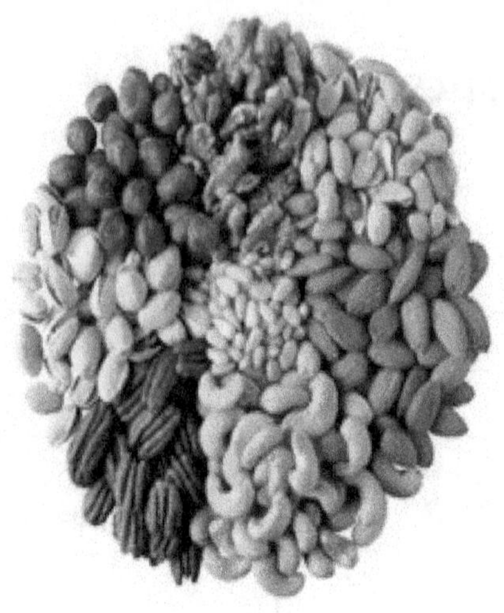

http://hatimicorporation.com/pictures/dry_fruits.jpg

Fresh fruits and vegetables

Fruits and vegetables are a fundamental component of any healthy and balanced diet. They provide the essential nutrients crucial to healthy living. Fruits such as Papaya have been known to reduce inflammation due to the presence of a chemical substance *bromelain*. This enzyme is also used in anti-inflammatory drug synthesis hence proving its benefits in the treatment of inflammation. Green vegetables such as broccoli are also a good remedy. It contains the phytonutrient sulforaphane which has anti-inflammatory properties. Similarly, sweet potato is a great source of vitamin B6, beta carotene and managansese which are all anti-oxidants and they work in harmony to fight inflammation in the body.

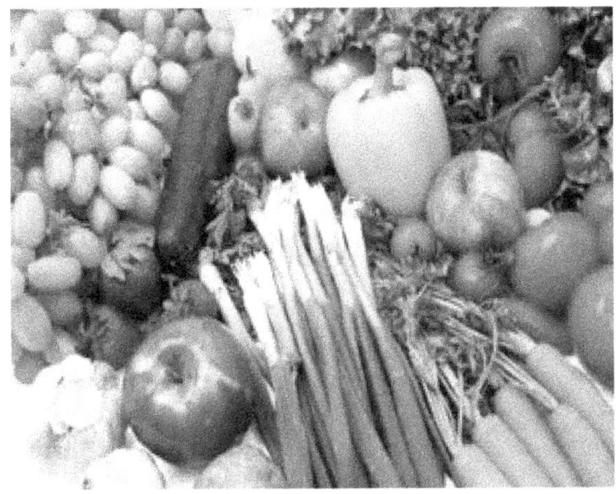

http://www.maximumworks.com/demo/commons/images/stories/pantry/veggie.jpg

Water

Last but not the least, water is one of the most effective way to heal and soothe inflammatory responses in the body. Not only is it vital for each and every metabolic reaction that occurs in the body but is also very beneficial in terms of flushing out and getting rid of harmful toxins from the body hence soothing inflammation.

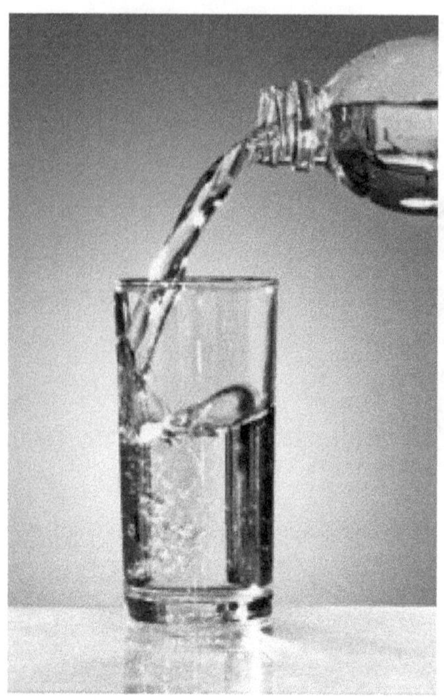

http://static.progressivemediagroup.com/uploads/imagelibrary/nri/water/ news/Mar%202012/water-drinking.JPG

What to avoid?

While it is very important to add beneficial foods to your diet that help the body in process of healing from inflammation, it is of equal and prime importance to avoid foods that cause and promote inflammation.

Deadly P's

The worst thing you can do to your body while it's trying to recover from inflammation is ingesting processed, packaged and prepared foods. These not only have high amounts of sugar and harmful carbs in them but are also packed with nasty additives that wreck your body by promoting inflammation.

Trans fats

These are abundant in goods found at the bakery. Momentarily, they tantalize your taste buds but in the long run wreak havoc for your body. Other sources include products made from margarine, deep fried items, and fast foods.

White sugars and Desserts

Any processed food, as mentioned earlier, is bad for your health. Desserts contain a large amount of complex carbohydrates and sugar as their chief ingredient which when taken in large amounts triggers the inflammation process of the digestive tract.

Chapter 4 – Specific Body Infections and Remedies for Treatment

During the course of our daily life we come across millions and millions of disease causing microbes such as bacteria, viruses and fungi. If it had not been for the body's immune system, we would contract diseases and infections from every single microbe through air, food and even water.

Even despite of the presence of body's natural defense, some powerful microbes are able to breach our immunity and invade the cells in the body causing infection. Antibiotics are the usual course of action when it comes to treating infections. However, antibiotics house in themselves myriad side effects and are also known to lower the natural immune response of the body, making the body dependent on antibiotics for minor infections as well as more susceptible to infections in the future. That's the bad news. The good news is that there are a number of natural preventive measures and remedies that can be undertaken in order to avoid the use of unnecessary medication and also naturally aid the treatment of infections.

Infections can commonly be divided into two broad categories;

- Bacterial infections

- Viral Infections

The microbes belonging to these two kingdoms are common infection causing agents and are known to cause hundreds of different kinds of infection in humans. Natural remedies have been seen to be strongly effective in the treatment and management of these infections. Discussed below are some items that can be employed in order to treat infection naturally.

Plant based remedies

Plants are the powerhouse of our planet. They are a great source of countless nutrients that benefit all mankind. Since the dawn of humanity, plant products have been used in the treatment of infectious diseases. The table below elaborates some examples of plant products along with the type of infection they inhibit and their respective individual benefit.

Table 4. Plant products and their uses in the treatment of bacterial and viral infections

Plant product	Bacterial/Viral	Type of Infection	Uses
Olive leaf	Viral	All types	Contains *oleuropein* which destroys viral cells, inhibits viral growth
Aloe vera	Bacterial	Urinary tract infections, skin infections	Used to treat internal infections such as UTI, Soothes and heals skin infections
Turmeric	Bacterial	Skin, respiratory infection	Rich in antioxidants. Protects against and fights bacterial infection. Promotes immunity
Tea tree oil	Viral and Bacterial	Respiratory, bladder infections	Used for treating chronic infection. Destroys bacterial and viral cells

Probiotics

Probiotics such as yogurt and fermented cheeses and vinegar are a great way of introducing good bacteria in your body. Intake of probiotic increases the population of healthy bacteria which fights and diminishes the harmful, disease causing bacteria hence preventing and treating present infections of the digestive tract.

Herbal and Spice Teas

Herbal teas are highly beneficial for aiding in the treatment of bacterial and viral infections alike. There are a lot of ways to incorporate healthy and beneficial herbs into your diet and using them as herbal teas is probably the most pleasing to taste buds. Here, we will discuss the benefits and uses of some herbal infusions that aid the treatment of viral and bacterial infections.

- *Cinnamon tea*

  This tasteful, anti-bacterial spice is used in tea as infusion, added to your diet or taken as a supplement. When taken as warm tea, it is known to boost immunity, aid digestion and diminish bacterial growth.

- *Ginger tea*

  Ginger is a powerful anti-bacteria agent. It is used to prevent and treat common cold caused by bacterial infection. With a drop of honey, this particular tea can do wonders for the common cold and flu infections.

- *Licorice root tea*

  It is known for its antibacterial and antiviral capabilities. Licorice has been seen to destroy the bacteria *H. pylori* that causes gastric ulcers and other stomach infections.

- *Clove tea*

Clove is a spice with a very strong and pleasant aroma and flavor. It is typically used as topical pain killer but is also extremely effective against bacterial infections that affect the intestine.

- *Sage tea*

Many plants of the mint family are used as remedies to counter infections of the respiratory tract. Sage tea is a very useful remedy for treatment of sore throat.

- *Mint, thyme and oregano*

These herbs, also belonging to the mint family contain *thymol* which is known antiseptic. They possess decongesting and expectorant which means that they breakdown the mucus in the respiratory tract which is a problem in lung and respiratory infections. The simplest way to use these herbs for infection remedy is to boil them for a short while in water and then inhale the steam so as to clear up the congestion.

Chapter 5 – Foods to Increase your Mind Power

A fully functional brain is the most integral part of any organism as it serves as the principle control center for all the mechanisms and activities of the body. Statistics show that owing to today's stressful and fast paced lifestyle, every single individual in today's world is at a higher risk of brain degenerative disorder as compared to 50 years ago. As our age progresses, the chances of contracting brain degeneration becomes significantly elevated. So evidently common sense implies that we do everything possible to maintain brain health. The healthiest and safest way to promote a healthy brain is the use of a suitable diet. Incorporating foods in your diet that benefit brain function can largely reduce your risk of brain disease later in life, and is hence beneficial in the long run!

Natural Oils

Good oils such as organic, unprocessed, cold pressed coconut oil and extra virgin olive oil are both rich in anti-oxidants that facilitate the working of the functional unit of the brain, the neurons, and also enhance brain function by counteracting free radicals that damage brain cells. Coconut oil is also a great source of saturated fats commonly referred to as "healthy fats". These healthy fats are a crucial nutrient required to achieve proper brain cell functioning. Avocado oil rich in monosaturated fatty acids has been shown to protect brain cells against damage.

Omega-3 Fatty Acids

A great source for obtaining omega-3 fatty acids is wild salmon. The omega-3 oi DHA present in salmon promotes brain health by stimulating the growth of brain cells and improving and retaining memory.

Berries

Berries such as blue berries and strawberries are known to be packed with powerful anti-oxidants that promote brain health. Blueberries also soothe inflammation which is a prime problem associated with brain degenerative disorders.

Nuts and Seeds

Walnuts and almonds in particular boost brain health as they are rich in anti-oxidants and brain friendly vitamin E complex. They are also known to improve memory. Seeds are also a powerhouse packed with highly beneficial nutrients and minerals. For instance, pumpkin seeds are a rich source of the micronutrient zinc which promotes memory and brain function.

Vitamins and Minerals

Vegetables like kale, spinach and broccoli are rich sources of vitamins C, K, A, folate as well as minerals like potassium and iron. These nutrients although required in low amounts by the body but are crucial to proper function. They help the brain fight against free radicals that damages nerve cells which in turn affects memory.

Tomatoes

Brightly colored and juicy, fresh tomatoes are rich in lycopene. Evidence suggests that due to the presence of this substance tomatoes could provide effective protection against free radicals in the brain that lead to neurodegenerative disorders like Alzheimer's disease and dementia.

Healthy Carbohydrates

Whole wheat and oatmeal when taken in unprocessed form can prove to be very beneficial for brain health. Studies show that people who start the day by taking whole grains for breakfast are far more likely to perform well throughout the day. Providing the brain with healthy carbohydrates ensures healthy brain function.

Iron rich foods

Scientific evidence suggests that even a low key iron deficiency in adults or children can have a large impact on cognitive function. Women and children are more to iron deficiency but fortunately reversal is possible with proper intake of a suitable diet. Foods in rich in iron are meat, fish, chicken, beans and soya beans among others.

Hydration

While it is of utter importance to stay hydrated by regularizing water intake, a very smart way of staying hydrated is including water rich foods in your diets. Try incorporating fruits like watermelon, cucumbers and salad greens in your diet. These have large reserves of water in them which helps keep the brain sharp by regulating flow of oxygen to the brain cells.

Chapter 6 – Exercise to boost immunity

How does it work?

It is a widely accepted fact that regular physical exertion has been proven to promote health in general. Studies have been conducted to exhibit the effect of exercise on the health of an individual. Evidence suggests that people who consistently employ exercise in their routine are far healthier compared to those who choose a lazy lifestyle. This is based on the principle that physical exertion boosts metabolism hence making digestion easier. The body utilizes the nutrients during exercise which results in less buildup of calories.

Apart from promoting general mental well-being and physical health, exercise has also been seen to boost immunity. This becomes possible in the following way.

- Physical exertion stimulates sweat glands to produce sweat. The excretion of sweat from the body also implies that harmful toxins will be flushed out from the body. It also helps the body get rid of harmful bacteria that otherwise maybe causative of infection. This in turn improves the body's natural defense.

- Secondly, exercise works to fluctuate the levels of white blood cells in the bossy. It makes it possible to improve blood circulation which makes the white blood cells move around the body at greater speed hence making microbe detection efficient and faster.

- Moreover, physical exertion, however gentle, results in a slight rise in the temperature of the body. This rise in temperature makes it difficult for bacterial growth to occur. It halts bacterial growth by changing the optimal temperature required for promoting bacterial growth.

- Exercising results in release of serotonin and oxytocin both of which are responsible for making a person feel mentally content and satisfied.

Sample routine

Gentle exercise like Yoga, Pilates and meditation have been known to improve the workings of the lymphatic system as well as circulation hence improving immunity. Below is a tabular and graphic representation of a few sample exercises that you can use to start yourself up.

Table 5. Types, demonstration and benefits of certain yoga steps

Type of exercise	Benefit	Demonstration
Cobra and Bridges	Provides strength to spine activating thymus gland which is a crucial organ for proper functioning of immune response.	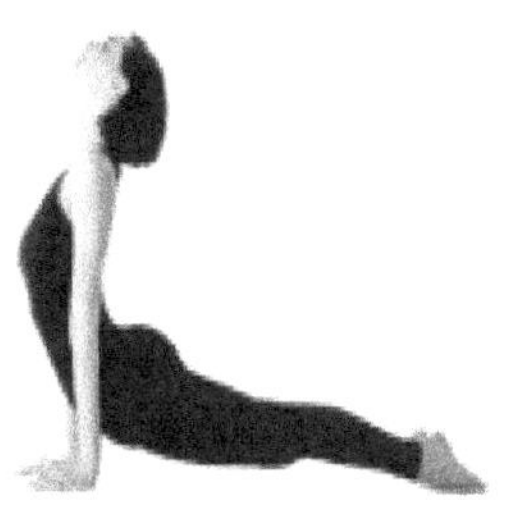 http://www.yogamagazine.com/wp-content/uploads/2012/04/Frog-Cobra-300x214.jpg
Shoulder stands, Ploughs	Evens out the distribution of immune cells through the body hence making immune response efficient.	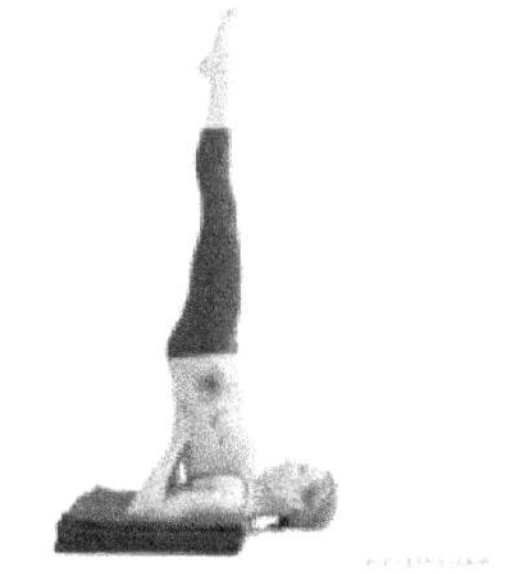 http://media.yogajournal.com/wp-content/uploads/supportedshoulderstandpose.jpg
Downward Dog	Relieves chronic respiratory congestion, improves immunity by improving circulation.	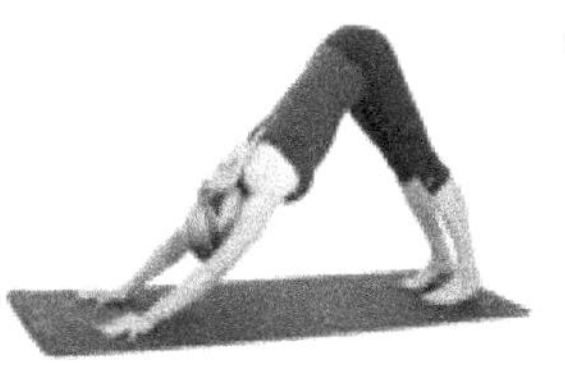 http://www.doyouyoga.com/wp-content/uploads/2016/01/downward-facing-dog-300x200.jpg

Word of Caution

Although exercise is a widely popular and accepted way of maintain physical and mental well-being, it is also important to keep in mind the fact that moderation is highly advisable. Excess of everything is bad. Make sure to learn proper techniques, start slow and be careful. While performing advanced level or extreme moves ensure that you have supervision of a licensed yoga therapist available.

Conclusion

Health is not the kind of thing that once can repurchase. Life is given to us once. We should take all measures possibly necessary to ensure a healthy lifestyle. In today's modern age, a common oversight is to ignore the power of natural and organic ways. People are regularly seen to opt for medicine for the treatment of problems ranging in complexity from simple to complicated, instead of turning towards natural preventive remedies and treatments which in the long run prove to be more beneficial. What people fail to realize is that your kitchen is the equivalent of a medical store, in fact only better! The foods and measures that we have discussed in this book are all commonly available all around the world and we can use them to our great advantage. These common items and simple exercises can be easily adjusted into your daily diet as preventive measures before counteracting any of the problems discussed and can also be used for treatment after the onset of the problem as is explicitly discussed in the chapters of this book. All the things discussed in the book cast light on the importance of incorporating natural foods wherever possible so as to avoid problems presently as well as later in life.

After reading this book you will be able to tackle problems regarding inflammation, immunity and brain from the comfort of your own home, naturally and without any harmful side effects. Also, you may incorporate light workout into your routine to ensure health and well-being. You are now better equipped to take care of your own health and of your loved ones around you. As they say, health is the greatest gift of all!

FREE Bonus Reminder

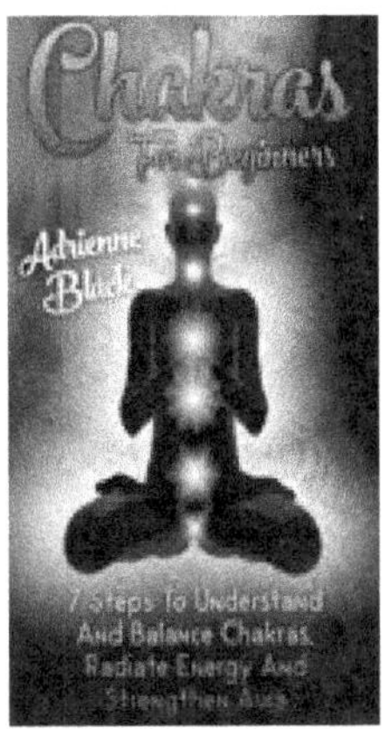

If you have not grabbed it yet, please go ahead and download your special bonus E book *"Chakras for Beginners. 7 Steps To Understand And Balance Chakras, Radiate Energy, And Strengthen Aura"*.

Simply Click the Button Below

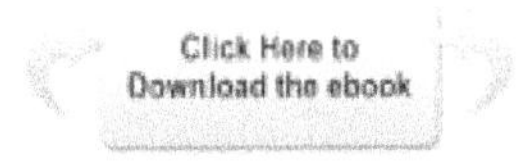

OR **Go to This Page**

http://lifehacksworld.com/free

BONUS #2: More Free & Discounted Books

Do you want to receive more Free & Discounted Books?

We have a mailing list where we send out our new Books when they go free or with a discount on Kindle. Click on the link below to sign up for Free & Discount Book Promotions.

=> Sign Up for Free & Discount Book Promotions <=

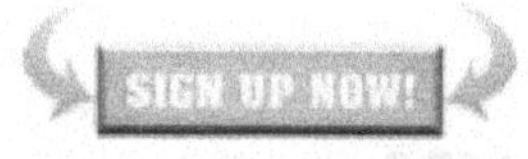

OR Go to this URL

http://zbit.ly/1WBb1Ek